VEGETARIAN SJOGREN SYNDROME DIET COOKBOOK FOR SENIORS

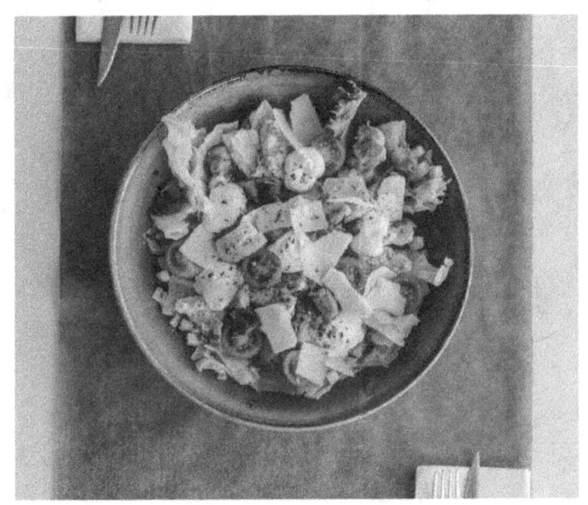

DR. JESSICA SMITH

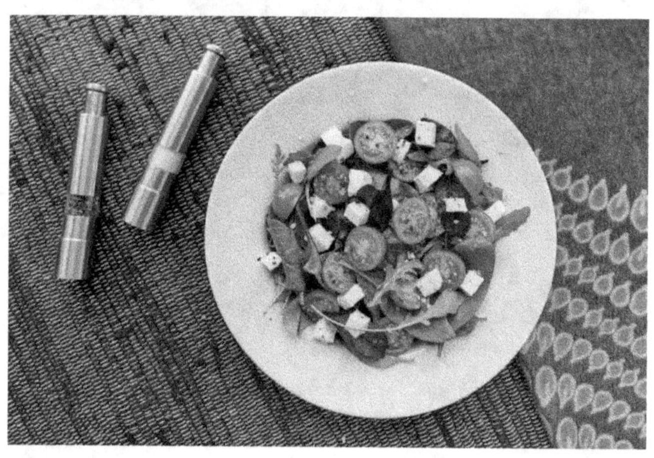

TABLE OF CONTENT

CHAPTER ONE

Understand the Vegetarian Sjogren Syndrome Diet:

Familiarize yourself with the basics of a vegetarian diet suitable for managing Sjogren's syndrome. Focus on incorporating plant-based proteins, healthy fats, and a variety of fruits and vegetables rich in antioxidants.

Consult with a Dietitian:

Before making any significant dietary changes, consult with a registered dietitian who can help tailor a meal plan to your specific needs as a senior with Sjogren's syndrome.

Stock Up on Sjogren-Friendly Foods:

Ensure your pantry is stocked with foods that are beneficial for managing Sjogren's symptoms, such as omega-3 rich seeds (flaxseeds, chia seeds), hydrating fruits (watermelon, cucumber), and calcium-fortified plant milks.

Plan Balanced Meals:

Aim to include a variety of nutrients in each meal to support overall health and symptom management.

Build meals around whole grains, legumes, leafy greens, and colorful vegetables.

Stay Hydrated:

Hydration is crucial for managing Sjogren's syndrome symptoms. Incorporate hydrating foods like soups, smoothies, and herbal teas into your daily diet, and aim to drink plenty of water throughout the day.

Experiment with Flavorful Herbs and Spices:

Enhance the taste of vegetarian dishes without relying on excessive salt by experimenting with flavorful herbs and spices such as basil, turmeric, ginger, and cilantro.

Include Omega-3 Fatty Acids:

Omega-3 fatty acids have anti-inflammatory properties that can help alleviate symptoms of Sjogren's syndrome. Incorporate sources such as walnuts, flaxseeds, hemp seeds, and algae-based supplements into your diet.

Opt for Easy-to-Digest Options:

Seniors may have more sensitive digestive systems, so choose easily digestible vegetarian protein sources such as tofu, tempeh, lentils, and cooked beans over harder-to-digest options.

Prioritize Oral Health:

Sjogren's syndrome can impact oral health, so prioritize foods that support dental hygiene, such as crunchy fruits and vegetables like apples, carrots, and celery, which can help stimulate saliva production and aid in digestion.

Listen to Your Body:

Pay attention to how different foods affect your symptoms and adjust your diet accordingly. Keep a food diary to track any triggers or patterns, and don't hesitate to make further dietary adjustments with the guidance of your healthcare team.

Understanding Vegetarian Sjogren Syndrome Diet for Seniors

Understanding the Vegetarian Sjogren Syndrome Diet for seniors involves recognizing the unique dietary needs and challenges faced by individuals living with this autoimmune condition. Sjogren's syndrome primarily affects the glands responsible for producing saliva and tears, leading to symptoms such as dry mouth, dry eyes, and difficulty swallowing.

Adopting a vegetarian diet tailored to manage these symptoms can significantly improve seniors' quality of life by focusing on foods that support hydration, oral health, and overall well-being.

A vegetarian diet for Sjogren's syndrome seniors emphasizes the consumption of plant-based foods rich in antioxidants, omega-3 fatty acids, and essential nutrients.

These include fruits, vegetables, whole grains, legumes, nuts, seeds, and plant-based sources of protein such as tofu and tempeh. Hydrating foods like watermelon, cucumber, and soups are also crucial for managing dryness symptoms.

Moreover, seniors with Sjogren's syndrome should prioritize oral health by incorporating crunchy fruits and vegetables that stimulate saliva production and support dental hygiene.

Additionally, they may benefit from reducing their intake of foods high in sugar, refined carbohydrates, and processed ingredients, which can exacerbate inflammation and other symptoms associated with the condition.

Understanding and adhering to a well-balanced vegetarian diet tailored to the specific needs of seniors with Sjogren's syndrome can help alleviate symptoms, improve overall health, and enhance their quality of life.

Consulting with a healthcare provider or registered dietitian is essential for developing a personalized dietary plan that optimally supports their health and well-being.

Principles of Vegetarian Sjogren Syndrome Diet for Seniors

The principles of a vegetarian diet for seniors with Sjogren's syndrome revolve around addressing the unique challenges posed by the condition while promoting overall health and well-being. Here are the key principles:

Hydration Focus: Seniors with Sjogren's syndrome often struggle with dry mouth and eyes due to reduced saliva and tear production.

Therefore, the diet emphasizes hydrating foods like water-rich fruits (e.g., watermelon, oranges) and vegetables (e.g., cucumber, celery), as well as soups and herbal teas to maintain adequate hydration levels.

Nutrient-Rich Foods: The diet prioritizes nutrient-dense plant-based foods such as fruits, vegetables, whole grains, legumes, nuts, and seeds.

These provide essential vitamins, minerals, antioxidants, and phytonutrients to support overall health and bolster the immune system.

Omega-3 Fatty Acids: Incorporating sources of omega-3 fatty acids, such as flaxseeds, chia seeds, walnuts, and algae-based supplements, can help reduce inflammation and alleviate symptoms associated with Sjogren's syndrome.

Oral Health Support: Since Sjogren's syndrome can lead to dental issues, the diet includes crunchy fruits and vegetables like apples, carrots, and bell peppers, which stimulate saliva production and aid in maintaining oral health.

Whole, Unprocessed Foods: Minimizing processed foods and refined sugars is key to reducing inflammation and supporting overall health. Instead, the focus is on whole, unprocessed plant-based foods to provide optimal nutrition.

Consultation with Healthcare Professionals: Seniors with Sjogren's syndrome should consult with healthcare professionals, including registered dietitians, to tailor the diet to their specific needs and ensure it complements their overall treatment plan.

Benefits of Vegetarian Sjogren Syndrome Diet for Seniors

The vegetarian diet tailored for seniors with Sjogren's syndrome offers numerous benefits that can significantly improve their overall health and well-being:

Reduced Inflammation: A plant-based diet rich in fruits, vegetables, whole grains, and legumes is naturally anti-inflammatory, which can help alleviate symptoms associated with Sjogren's syndrome, such as joint pain and fatigue.

Hydration Support: Hydrating foods like water-rich fruits and vegetables, as well as soups and herbal teas, help seniors with Sjogren's syndrome combat dry mouth and eyes, supporting better overall hydration.

Nutrient-Rich: Plant-based foods are abundant in essential vitamins, minerals, antioxidants, and phytonutrients, which are crucial for supporting immune function, improving energy levels, and promoting overall health in seniors.

Heart Health: By focusing on plant-based sources of protein and healthy fats, such as nuts, seeds, and legumes, the vegetarian diet can help seniors maintain healthy cholesterol levels and reduce the risk of cardiovascular disease.

Improved Digestion: Seniors often experience digestive issues, and a vegetarian diet rich in fiber from fruits, vegetables, and whole grains can promote regular bowel movements, alleviate constipation, and support gastrointestinal health.

Weight Management: Plant-based diets tend to be lower in calories and saturated fats while being higher in fiber, which can help seniors manage their weight more effectively and reduce the risk of obesity-related conditions.

Enhanced Oral Health: Incorporating crunchy fruits and vegetables into the diet stimulates saliva production, helping seniors maintain better oral hygiene and reducing the risk of dental issues associated with Sjogren's syndrome.

Adopting a vegetarian diet tailored to seniors with Sjogren's syndrome requires careful consideration and planning. Here are some essential tips to help navigate this dietary approach effectively:

Hydration is Key: Seniors with Sjogren's syndrome should prioritize hydrating foods such as water-rich fruits (watermelon, oranges) and vegetables (cucumber, celery) to combat dry mouth and eyes. Soups, herbal teas, and coconut water can also contribute to hydration.

Focus on Nutrient Density: Ensure the diet includes a variety of nutrient-dense foods like fruits, vegetables, whole grains, legumes, nuts, and seeds to provide essential vitamins, minerals, and antioxidants necessary for overall health and symptom management.

Omega-3 Fatty Acids: Incorporate plant-based sources of omega-3 fatty acids such as flaxseeds, chia seeds, walnuts, and algae-based supplements to help reduce inflammation and alleviate symptoms associated with Sjogren's syndrome.

Opt for Easy-to-Digest Proteins: Seniors may benefit from easily digestible protein sources like tofu, tempeh, lentils, and cooked beans, which can help prevent digestive discomfort and support muscle health.

Hygiene and Dental Health: Include crunchy fruits and vegetables like apples, carrots, and bell peppers in the diet to stimulate saliva production and aid in maintaining oral hygiene. Regular dental check-ups are essential for preventing dental issues.

Reduce Inflammatory Foods: Minimize intake of processed foods, refined sugars, and saturated fats, which can exacerbate inflammation and worsen symptoms. Focus on whole, unprocessed plant-based foods instead.

Consult with a Healthcare Professional: Seek guidance from a registered dietitian or healthcare provider to tailor the vegetarian diet to individual needs, ensuring it complements treatment and supports overall health effectively.

By following these tips, seniors with Sjogren's syndrome can create a balanced and nourishing vegetarian diet that helps manage symptoms, supports hydration, promotes oral health, and enhances overall well-being.

Guidelines for a vegetarian diet tailored to seniors with Sjogren's syndrome provide a structured approach to managing symptoms and promoting overall health. Here are essential guidelines to follow:

Hydration: Prioritize hydration by consuming water-rich fruits and vegetables, herbal teas, and soups to combat dry mouth and eyes, common symptoms of Sjogren's syndrome.

Nutrient-Rich Foods: Emphasize a variety of nutrient-dense plant-based foods, including fruits, vegetables, whole grains, legumes, nuts, and seeds, to provide essential vitamins, minerals, and antioxidants.

Omega-3 Fatty Acids: Incorporate plant-based sources of omega-3 fatty acids, such as flaxseeds, chia seeds, walnuts, and algae-based supplements, to help reduce inflammation and alleviate symptoms.

Protein Sources: Choose easily digestible protein sources like tofu, tempeh, lentils, and cooked beans to support muscle health without exacerbating digestive discomfort.

Oral Health Support: Include crunchy fruits and vegetables like apples, carrots, and celery to stimulate saliva production and maintain oral hygiene, reducing the risk of dental issues associated with Sjogren's syndrome.

Limit Inflammatory Foods: Minimize intake of processed foods, refined sugars, and saturated fats, as they can worsen inflammation and exacerbate symptoms.

Consultation with Healthcare Professionals: Seek guidance from a registered dietitian or healthcare provider to personalize the diet plan according to individual needs, ensuring it complements treatment and supports overall well-being effectively.

By adhering to these guidelines, seniors with Sjogren's syndrome can create a balanced and nourishing vegetarian diet that helps manage symptoms, promotes hydration, supports oral health, and enhances overall quality of life.

CHAPTER TWO

Vegetarian Sjogren Syndrome Diet Breakfast Recipes

1: Chia Seed Pudding

Ingredients:

- ➤ 2 tablespoons chia seeds
- ➤ 1/2 cup plant-based milk (almond, soy, coconut)
- ➤ 1/2 teaspoon vanilla extract
- ➤ Fresh berries for topping

Instructions:

- ➤ In a bowl, mix chia seeds, plant-based milk, and vanilla extract. Stir well.
- ➤ Refrigerate overnight or for at least 2 hours until it thickens.
- ➤ Serve topped with fresh berries.

Health Benefits:

- ➤ Chia seeds are rich in omega-3 fatty acids, fiber, and antioxidants, which help reduce inflammation and support heart health.

Preparation Time: 5 minutes (+ chilling time)

2: Berry Smoothie Bowl

Ingredients:

- ➢ 1 cup mixed berries (strawberries, blueberries, raspberries)
- ➢ 1/2 banana
- ➢ 1/2 cup spinach
- ➢ 1/2 cup plant-based yogurt
- ➢ 1 tablespoon chia seeds (optional)
- ➢ Granola for topping

Instructions:

- ➢ Blend mixed berries, banana, spinach, plant-based yogurt, and chia seeds until smooth.
- ➢ Pour into a bowl and top with granola.

Health Benefits:

- ➢ This smoothie bowl is packed with antioxidants, vitamins, and minerals from the berries and spinach, supporting immune function and overall health.

Preparation Time: 5 minutes

3: Avocado Toast

Ingredients:

- ➢ 1 ripe avocado
- ➢ 2 slices whole grain bread
- ➢ 1 tablespoon lemon juice
- ➢ Salt and pepper to taste
- ➢ Red pepper flakes for garnish (optional)

Instructions:

- ➢ Mash the avocado with lemon juice, salt, and pepper.
- ➢ Toast the bread slices until golden brown.
- ➢ Spread the mashed avocado on the toast and sprinkle with red pepper flakes if desired.

Health Benefits:

- ➢ Avocados are rich in healthy fats, vitamins, and minerals, promoting heart health and providing essential nutrients for seniors.

Preparation Time: 10 minutes

Ingredients:

- 1/2 cup rolled oats
- 1/2 cup plant-based milk
- 1 tablespoon maple syrup
- 1/2 teaspoon vanilla extract
- Sliced banana for topping

Instructions:

- In a jar, combine rolled oats, plant-based milk, maple syrup, and vanilla extract. Stir well.
- Refrigerate overnight.
- In the morning, top with sliced banana before serving.

Health Benefits:

- Overnight oats are rich in fiber, vitamins, and minerals, supporting digestion and providing sustained energy throughout the morning.

Preparation Time: 5 minutes (+ chilling time)

Ingredients:

- ➢ 1/2 block tofu, crumbled
- ➢ 1/4 cup diced bell peppers
- ➢ 1/4 cup diced onions
- ➢ 1/2 teaspoon turmeric powder
- ➢ Salt and pepper to taste
- ➢ Fresh parsley for garnish

Instructions:

- ➢ In a pan, sauté diced bell peppers and onions until softened.
- ➢ Add crumbled tofu and turmeric powder. Cook until heated through.
- ➢ Season with salt and pepper, and garnish with fresh parsley before serving.

Health Benefits:

- ➢ Tofu is a great source of plant-based protein, while bell peppers and onions provide antioxidants and vitamins, supporting immune function.

Preparation Time: 15 minutes

6: Veggie Omelette

Ingredients:

- 2 eggs (or tofu for a vegan option)
- 1/4 cup diced tomatoes
- 1/4 cup chopped spinach
- 1 tablespoon diced onions
- Salt and pepper to taste
- 1 teaspoon olive oil

Instructions:

- In a bowl, whisk eggs with salt and pepper.
- Heat olive oil in a pan over medium heat.
- Add diced tomatoes, chopped spinach, and diced onions to the pan. Cook until softened.
- Pour the whisked eggs over the veggies and cook until set.
- Fold the omelette in half and serve.

Health Benefits:

- Eggs (or tofu) provide protein, while tomatoes and spinach offer vitamins and antioxidants, supporting overall health and immunity.

Preparation Time: 10 minutes

7: Quinoa Breakfast Bowl

Ingredients:

- 1/2 cup cooked quinoa
- 1/4 cup sliced almonds
- 1/4 cup diced apples
- 1 tablespoon maple syrup
- 1/2 teaspoon cinnamon
- Plant-based yogurt for topping

Instructions:

- In a bowl, combine cooked quinoa, sliced almonds, diced apples, maple syrup, and cinnamon. Mix well.
- Serve topped with plant-based yogurt.

Health Benefits:

- Quinoa is a complete protein, providing essential amino acids, while almonds and apples offer fiber, vitamins, and minerals, supporting digestive health.

Preparation Time: 15 minutes

8: Banana Walnut Pancakes

Ingredients:

- ➤ 1 ripe banana, mashed
- ➤ 1/2 cup whole wheat flour
- ➤ 1/2 cup plant-based milk
- ➤ 1/4 cup chopped walnuts
- ➤ 1 tablespoon maple syrup
- ➤ 1/2 teaspoon baking powder
- ➤ 1/2 teaspoon vanilla extract
- ➤ Pinch of salt
- ➤ Coconut oil for cooking

Instructions:

- ➤ In a bowl, mix mashed banana, whole wheat flour, plant-based milk, chopped walnuts, maple syrup, baking powder, vanilla extract, and salt until well combined.
- ➤ Heat coconut oil in a pan over medium heat.
- ➤ Pour batter onto the pan to form pancakes and cook until bubbles form on the surface.
- ➤ Flip and cook until golden brown on both sides.

> Serve with additional sliced bananas and maple syrup if desired.

Health Benefits:

> These pancakes are a nutritious and delicious breakfast option, providing fiber, protein, and healthy fats to support energy levels and overall health.

Preparation Time: 20 minutes

9: Spinach and Feta Frittata

Ingredients:

> 4 eggs
> 1/2 cup chopped spinach
> 1/4 cup crumbled feta cheese
> 1/4 cup diced tomatoes
> 1/4 cup diced onions
> Salt and pepper to taste
> 1 teaspoon olive oil

Instructions:

> Preheat the oven to 375°F (190°C).
> In a bowl, whisk eggs with salt and pepper.

- ➢ Heat olive oil in an oven-safe skillet over medium heat.
- ➢ Add diced tomatoes and onions to the skillet. Cook until softened.
- ➢ Add chopped spinach and cook until wilted.
- ➢ Pour the whisked eggs over the veggies and sprinkle crumbled feta cheese on top.
- ➢ Transfer the skillet to the oven and bake for 15-20 minutes or until the frittata is set.
- ➢ Slice and serve.

Health Benefits:

- ➢ Spinach is rich in vitamins and minerals, while eggs provide protein and essential nutrients, making this frittata a nutritious breakfast option for seniors.

Preparation Time: 30 minutes

10: Peanut Butter Banana Smoothie

Ingredients:

- ➢ 1 ripe banana
- ➢ 2 tablespoons peanut butter
- ➢ 1 cup plant-based milk

- ➢ 1 tablespoon honey or maple syrup (optional)
- ➢ Ice cubes

Instructions:

- ➢ In a blender, combine ripe banana, peanut butter, plant-based milk, honey or maple syrup (if using), and ice cubes.
- ➢ Blend until smooth and creamy.
- ➢ Pour into a glass and serve immediately.

Health Benefits:

- ➢ This smoothie is a satisfying and nutritious breakfast option, providing protein, healthy fats, and essential nutrients from peanut butter and banana.

Preparation Time: 5 minutes

Vegetarian Sjogren Syndrome Diet Lunch Recipes

1: Quinoa Salad

Ingredients:

- ➢ 1 cup cooked quinoa
- ➢ 1/2 cup chopped cucumber

- 1/2 cup diced tomatoes
- 1/4 cup chopped parsley
- 1/4 cup crumbled feta cheese
- 2 tablespoons olive oil
- 1 tablespoon lemon juice
- Salt and pepper to taste

Instructions:

- In a bowl, combine cooked quinoa, chopped cucumber, diced tomatoes, chopped parsley, and crumbled feta cheese.
- Drizzle with olive oil and lemon juice. Season with salt and pepper.
- Toss gently to combine and serve chilled.

Health Benefits:

- This quinoa salad is rich in protein, fiber, vitamins, and minerals, providing sustained energy and supporting overall health.

Preparation Time: 15 minutes

2: Lentil Soup

Ingredients:

- ➤ 1 cup dried green lentils
- ➤ 4 cups vegetable broth
- ➤ 1 onion, diced
- ➤ 2 carrots, diced
- ➤ 2 celery stalks, diced
- ➤ 2 cloves garlic, minced
- ➤ 1 teaspoon ground cumin
- ➤ 1 teaspoon ground coriander
- ➤ Salt and pepper to taste
- ➤ Fresh parsley for garnish

Instructions:

- ➤ In a large pot, combine dried lentils, vegetable broth, diced onion, carrots, celery, minced garlic, ground cumin, and ground coriander.
- ➤ Bring to a boil, then reduce heat and simmer for 20-25 minutes or until lentils are tender.
- ➤ Season with salt and pepper to taste.
- ➤ Serve hot, garnished with fresh parsley.

Health Benefits:

> ➤ Lentils are a good source of protein, fiber, and iron, while vegetables provide essential vitamins and minerals, supporting overall health and digestion.

Preparation Time: 30 minutes

3: Chickpea Salad Sandwich

Ingredients:

> ➤ 1 can (15 oz) chickpeas, drained and rinsed
> ➤ 1/4 cup diced celery
> ➤ 1/4 cup diced red onion
> ➤ 2 tablespoons chopped fresh dill
> ➤ 2 tablespoons lemon juice
> ➤ 2 tablespoons vegan mayonnaise
> ➤ Salt and pepper to taste
> ➤ Whole grain bread slices
> ➤ Lettuce leaves and tomato slices for serving

Instructions:

> ➤ In a bowl, mash chickpeas with a fork until slightly chunky.

- ➢ Add diced celery, red onion, chopped fresh dill, lemon juice, vegan mayonnaise, salt, and pepper. Stir well to combine.
- ➢ Spread chickpea salad onto whole grain bread slices.
- ➢ Top with lettuce leaves, tomato slices, and another slice of bread to make a sandwich.
- ➢ Cut in half and serve.

Health Benefits:

- ➢ Chickpeas are rich in protein and fiber, while vegetables provide vitamins and antioxidants, making this sandwich a nutritious lunch option for seniors.

Preparation Time: 15 minutes

4: Vegetable Stir-Fry

Ingredients:

- ➢ 2 cups mixed vegetables (bell peppers, broccoli, carrots, snap peas)
- ➢ 1/2 cup tofu, cubed
- ➢ 2 tablespoons soy sauce (or tamari for gluten-free option)

- ➢ 1 tablespoon sesame oil
- ➢ 2 cloves garlic, minced
- ➢ 1 teaspoon grated ginger
- ➢ Cooked brown rice for serving

Instructions:

- ➢ Heat sesame oil in a large pan or wok over medium heat.
- ➢ Add minced garlic and grated ginger. Cook for 1 minute until fragrant.
- ➢ Add mixed vegetables and tofu cubes to the pan. Stir-fry for 5-7 minutes until vegetables are tender-crisp.
- ➢ Stir in soy sauce and cook for another 1-2 minutes.
- ➢ Serve over cooked brown rice.

Health Benefits:

- ➢ This vegetable stir-fry is packed with fiber, vitamins, and antioxidants from the mixed vegetables and tofu, supporting digestive health and overall well-being.

Preparation Time: 20 minutes

5: Mediterranean Wrap

Ingredients:

- ➢ 1 whole wheat tortilla
- ➢ 2 tablespoons hummus
- ➢ 1/4 cup chopped cucumber
- ➢ 1/4 cup diced tomatoes
- ➢ 2 tablespoons crumbled feta cheese
- ➢ 1 tablespoon chopped kalamata olives
- ➢ Fresh spinach leaves

Instructions:

- ➢ Spread hummus evenly over the whole wheat tortilla.
- ➢ Layer chopped cucumber, diced tomatoes, crumbled feta cheese, chopped kalamata olives, and fresh spinach leaves on top.
- ➢ Roll up the tortilla tightly to form a wrap.
- ➢ Cut in half and serve.

Health Benefits:

- ➢ This Mediterranean wrap is a flavorful and nutritious lunch option, providing protein, fiber, and essential nutrients from the vegetables, hummus, and feta cheese.

Preparation Time: 10 minutes

6: Black Bean Quesadilla

Ingredients:

- 2 whole grain tortillas
- 1/2 cup canned black beans, drained and rinsed
- 1/4 cup diced bell peppers
- 1/4 cup diced onions
- 1/2 cup shredded cheese (vegan cheese for a vegan option)
- Salsa and guacamole for serving

Instructions:

- Heat a non-stick skillet over medium heat.
- Place one whole grain tortilla in the skillet. Layer with black beans, diced bell peppers, onions, and shredded cheese. Top with another tortilla.
- Cook for 2-3 minutes on each side until the tortilla is golden brown and the cheese is melted.
- Cut into wedges and serve with salsa and guacamole.

Health Benefits:

> ➢ Black beans are rich in protein and fiber, while bell peppers and onions provide vitamins and antioxidants, making this quesadilla a satisfying and nutritious lunch option for seniors.

Preparation Time: 15 minutes

7: Spinach and Mushroom Quiche

Ingredients:

> ➢ 1 prepared whole wheat pie crust
> ➢ 2 cups fresh spinach leaves
> ➢ 1 cup sliced mushrooms
> ➢ 1/2 cup diced onions
> ➢ 4 eggs (or tofu for a vegan option)
> ➢ 1 cup plant-based milk
> ➢ 1/2 cup shredded cheese (optional)
> ➢ Salt and pepper to taste
> ➢ Olive oil for cooking

Instructions:

> ➢ Preheat the oven to 375°F (190°C).

- ➢ Heat olive oil in a skillet over medium heat. Add sliced mushrooms and diced onions. Cook until softened.
- ➢ Add fresh spinach leaves to the skillet and cook until wilted.
- ➢ In a bowl, whisk eggs with plant-based milk, salt, and pepper.
- ➢ Spread the cooked vegetables evenly in the prepared whole wheat pie crust.
- ➢ Pour the egg mixture over the vegetables. Sprinkle shredded cheese on top if using.
- ➢ Bake in the preheated oven for 30-35 minutes or until the quiche is set and golden brown.
- ➢ Allow to cool slightly before slicing and serving.

Health Benefits:

- ➢ Spinach and mushrooms are rich in vitamins, minerals, and antioxidants, while eggs (or tofu) provide protein and essential nutrients, making this quiche a nutritious and delicious lunch option for seniors.

Preparation Time: 45 minutes

8: Caprese Salad

Ingredients:

- ➤ 1 cup cherry tomatoes, halved
- ➤ 1/2 cup fresh mozzarella balls
- ➤ 1/4 cup fresh basil leaves, torn
- ➤ 1 tablespoon balsamic vinegar
- ➤ 1 tablespoon extra virgin olive oil
- ➤ Salt and pepper to taste

Instructions:

- ➤ In a bowl, combine halved cherry tomatoes, fresh mozzarella balls, and torn basil leaves.
- ➤ Drizzle with balsamic vinegar and extra virgin olive oil.
- ➤ Season with salt and pepper to taste.
- ➤ Toss gently to combine and serve.

Health Benefits:

- ➤ This Caprese salad is a simple and refreshing lunch option, providing vitamins, minerals, and healthy fats from the tomatoes, mozzarella, and olive oil.

Preparation Time: 10 minutes

9: Sweet Potato and Black Bean Burrito Bowl

Ingredients:

> - 1 cup cooked quinoa
> - 1 cup cooked black beans
> - 1 small sweet potato, roasted and cubed
> - 1/2 avocado, sliced
> - 1/4 cup salsa
> - 1/4 cup chopped cilantro
> - Lime wedges for serving

Instructions:

> - Divide cooked quinoa, black beans, roasted sweet potato cubes, sliced avocado, salsa, and chopped cilantro among serving bowls.
> - Serve with lime wedges on the side for squeezing over the bowl.

Health Benefits:

> - This burrito bowl is packed with fiber, protein, vitamins, and minerals from the quinoa, black beans, sweet potato, and avocado, providing sustained energy and supporting overall health.

Preparation Time: 30 minutes

10: Vegetable and Bean Soup

Ingredients:

- 4 cups vegetable broth
- 1 can (15 oz) diced tomatoes
- 1 cup chopped carrots
- 1 cup chopped celery
- 1 cup chopped zucchini
- 1 can (15 oz) kidney beans, drained and rinsed
- 1 teaspoon dried thyme
- 1 teaspoon dried oregano
- Salt and pepper to taste
- Fresh parsley for garnish

Instructions:

- In a large pot, combine vegetable broth, diced tomatoes, chopped carrots, chopped celery, chopped zucchini, kidney beans, dried thyme, and dried oregano.
- Bring to a boil, then reduce heat and simmer for 20-25 minutes or until vegetables are tender.
- Season with salt and pepper to taste.

> Serve hot, garnished with fresh parsley.

Health Benefits:

> This vegetable and bean soup is rich in fiber, vitamins, and minerals, providing immune support and promoting digestive health for seniors.

Preparation Time: 30 minutes

Vegetarian Sjogren Syndrome Diet Dinner Recipes

1: Lentil Soup

Ingredients:

> 1 cup dried green lentils
> 4 cups vegetable broth
> 1 onion, diced
> 2 carrots, diced
> 2 celery stalks, diced
> 2 cloves garlic, minced
> 1 teaspoon ground cumin
> 1 teaspoon ground turmeric
> Salt and pepper to taste
> Fresh parsley for garnish

Instructions:

> - In a large pot, sauté diced onion, carrots, and celery until softened.
> - Add minced garlic, ground cumin, and ground turmeric. Cook for 1-2 minutes until fragrant.
> - Rinse lentils under cold water and add them to the pot along with vegetable broth.
> - Bring to a boil, then reduce heat and simmer for 20-25 minutes until lentils are tender.
> - Season with salt and pepper to taste.
> - Garnish with fresh parsley before serving.

Health Benefits:

> - Lentils are rich in protein, fiber, and iron, providing essential nutrients for seniors with Sjogren's syndrome.

Preparation Time: 30 minutes

2: Vegetable Stir-Fry

Ingredients:

> - 2 cups mixed vegetables (bell peppers, broccoli, carrots, snap peas)

- ➤ 1/2 block tofu, cubed
- ➤ 2 tablespoons soy sauce
- ➤ 1 tablespoon sesame oil
- ➤ 2 cloves garlic, minced
- ➤ 1 teaspoon grated ginger
- ➤ Cooked brown rice for serving

Instructions:

- ➤ Heat sesame oil in a large skillet or wok over medium-high heat.
- ➤ Add minced garlic and grated ginger, and sauté for 1 minute until fragrant.
- ➤ Add cubed tofu and cook until lightly browned on all sides.
- ➤ Add mixed vegetables to the skillet and stir-fry until tender-crisp.
- ➤ Pour soy sauce over the vegetables and tofu, and toss to coat evenly.
- ➤ Serve over cooked brown rice.

Health Benefits:

> This vegetable stir-fry is packed with vitamins, minerals, and antioxidants, supporting immune function and overall health in seniors.

Preparation Time: 20 minutes

3: Chickpea Curry

Ingredients:

> 1 can chickpeas, drained and rinsed

> 1 onion, diced

> 2 tomatoes, diced

> 2 cloves garlic, minced

> 1 tablespoon grated ginger

> 1 tablespoon curry powder

> 1 teaspoon ground cumin

> 1 teaspoon ground coriander

> 1/2 cup coconut milk

> Fresh cilantro for garnish

> Cooked quinoa or brown rice for serving

Instructions:

> In a large skillet, sauté diced onion until translucent.

- ➢ Add minced garlic and grated ginger, and cook for 1-2 minutes until fragrant.
- ➢ Stir in diced tomatoes, curry powder, ground cumin, and ground coriander.
- ➢ Add drained chickpeas to the skillet and cook for 5-7 minutes.
- ➢ Pour coconut milk over the chickpea mixture and simmer for another 5 minutes.
- ➢ Garnish with fresh cilantro and serve over cooked quinoa or brown rice.

Health Benefits:

- ➢ Chickpeas are a good source of protein and fiber, while coconut milk adds creaminess and healthy fats to this nutritious curry.

Preparation Time: 30 minutes

4: Vegetable Quinoa Bowl

Ingredients:

- ➢ 1 cup cooked quinoa
- ➢ 1 cup mixed roasted vegetables (zucchini, bell peppers, cherry tomatoes)

> 1/4 cup crumbled feta cheese

> 2 tablespoons balsamic glaze

> Fresh basil leaves for garnish

Instructions:

> In a bowl, layer cooked quinoa and mixed roasted vegetables.

> Sprinkle crumbled feta cheese on top.

> Drizzle balsamic glaze over the bowl.

> Garnish with fresh basil leaves before serving.

Health Benefits:

> This vegetable quinoa bowl is packed with fiber, vitamins, and minerals from quinoa and roasted vegetables, supporting digestive health and overall well-being.

Preparation Time: 20 minutes

5: Spinach and Mushroom Pasta

Ingredients:

> 8 oz whole wheat pasta

> 2 cups fresh spinach leaves

> 1 cup sliced mushrooms

➤ 2 cloves garlic, minced

➤ 2 tablespoons olive oil

➤ 1/4 cup grated Parmesan cheese (optional)

➤ Salt and pepper to taste

Instructions:

➤ Cook pasta according to package instructions until al dente. Drain and set aside.

➤ In a large skillet, heat olive oil over medium heat.

➤ Add minced garlic and sliced mushrooms to the skillet. Cook until mushrooms are tender.

➤ Add fresh spinach leaves to the skillet and cook until wilted.

➤ Toss cooked pasta with the spinach and mushroom mixture.

➤ Season with salt and pepper to taste.

➤ Sprinkle grated Parmesan cheese on top before serving if desired.

Health Benefits:

➤ Spinach and mushrooms are rich in vitamins, minerals, and antioxidants, while whole wheat pasta provides fiber and essential nutrients, making this dish a nutritious option for seniors.

Preparation Time: 20 minutes

6: Stuffed Bell Peppers

Ingredients:

- 4 large bell peppers, halved and seeded
- 1 cup cooked quinoa
- 1 can black beans, drained and rinsed
- 1 cup diced tomatoes
- 1/2 cup corn kernels
- 1/4 cup chopped cilantro
- 1 teaspoon ground cumin
- 1/2 teaspoon chili powder
- Salt and pepper to taste
- 1/2 cup shredded cheddar cheese (optional)

Instructions:

- Preheat the oven to 375°F (190°C).
- In a large bowl, mix cooked quinoa, black beans, diced tomatoes, corn kernels, chopped cilantro, ground cumin, chili powder, salt, and pepper.

- Stuff the halved bell peppers with the quinoa mixture.
- Place the stuffed bell peppers in a baking dish and cover with foil.
- Bake for 25-30 minutes until the peppers are tender.
- Remove the foil, sprinkle shredded cheddar cheese on top (if using), and bake for an additional 5 minutes until the cheese is melted and bubbly.
- Serve hot.

Health Benefits:

- Bell peppers are rich in vitamins and antioxidants, while quinoa and black beans provide protein, fiber, and essential nutrients, making this dish a nutritious and satisfying dinner option for seniors.

Preparation Time: 45 minutes

7: Veggie Burger

Ingredients:

- 1 can chickpeas, drained and rinsed
- 1/2 cup cooked quinoa
- 1/4 cup breadcrumbs

- ➢ 1/4 cup grated carrots
- ➢ 1/4 cup diced bell peppers
- ➢ 1/4 cup chopped spinach
- ➢ 2 cloves garlic, minced
- ➢ 1 teaspoon ground cumin
- ➢ 1/2 teaspoon smoked paprika
- ➢ Salt and pepper to taste
- ➢ Whole grain burger buns
- ➢ Lettuce, tomato slices, avocado slices for topping

Instructions:

- ➢ In a food processor, pulse chickpeas until coarsely mashed.
- ➢ In a large bowl, combine mashed chickpeas, cooked quinoa, breadcrumbs, grated carrots, diced bell peppers, chopped spinach, minced garlic, ground cumin, smoked paprika, salt, and pepper. Mix until well combined.
- ➢ Form the mixture into patties.
- ➢ Heat a non-stick skillet over medium heat and cook the veggie burgers for 3-4 minutes on each side until golden brown.

> Serve the veggie burgers on whole grain burger buns, topped with lettuce, tomato slices, and avocado slices.

Health Benefits:

> These veggie burgers are packed with plant-based protein, fiber, and essential nutrients, providing a nutritious and satisfying dinner option for seniors.

Preparation Time: 30 minutes

8: Eggplant Parmesan

Ingredients:

> 1 large eggplant, sliced into rounds
> 1 cup whole wheat breadcrumbs
> 1/2 cup grated Parmesan cheese
> 2 eggs, beaten (or flaxseed meal mixed with water for a vegan option)
> 2 cups marinara sauce
> 1/2 cup shredded mozzarella cheese
> Fresh basil leaves for garnish
> Olive oil for brushing

Instructions:

- ➢ Preheat the oven to 400°F (200°C). Line a baking sheet with parchment paper.
- ➢ In a shallow dish, combine whole wheat breadcrumbs and grated Parmesan cheese.
- ➢ Dip eggplant slices into beaten eggs (or flaxseed mixture), then coat with breadcrumb mixture.
- ➢ Place coated eggplant slices on the prepared baking sheet.
- ➢ Brush the tops of the eggplant slices with olive oil.
- ➢ Bake for 20-25 minutes until golden brown and crispy.
- ➢ In a baking dish, spread a layer of marinara sauce. Place baked eggplant slices on top.
- ➢ Top with remaining marinara sauce and shredded mozzarella cheese.
- ➢ Bake for an additional 15 minutes until the cheese is melted and bubbly.
- ➢ Garnish with fresh basil leaves before serving.

Health Benefits:

> ➤ Eggplant is a low-calorie vegetable rich in fiber and antioxidants, while whole wheat breadcrumbs provide added fiber and nutrients, making this dish a nutritious and delicious dinner option for seniors.

Preparation Time: 45 minutes

9: Lentil Shepherd's Pie

Ingredients:

> ➤ 1 cup dried green lentils
> ➤ 2 cups vegetable broth
> ➤ 1 onion, diced
> ➤ 2 carrots, diced
> ➤ 2 celery stalks, diced
> ➤ 2 cloves garlic, minced
> ➤ 1 teaspoon dried thyme
> ➤ 1 teaspoon dried rosemary
> ➤ Salt and pepper to taste
> ➤ Mashed potatoes for topping

Instructions:

> In a large pot, combine dried green lentils and vegetable broth. Bring to a boil, then reduce heat and simmer for 20-25 minutes until lentils are tender.

> In a skillet, sauté diced onion, carrots, and celery until softened.

> Add minced garlic, dried thyme, and dried rosemary to the skillet. Cook for 1-2 minutes until fragrant.

> Preheat the oven to 375°F (190°C).

> Combine cooked lentils and sautéed vegetables in a baking dish. Season with salt and pepper to taste.

> Spread mashed potatoes evenly over the lentil mixture.

> Bake for 25-30 minutes until the mashed potatoes are golden brown.

> Serve hot.

Health Benefits:

> Lentils are a good source of plant-based protein and fiber, while vegetables provide essential vitamins and minerals, making this dish a nutritious and comforting dinner option for seniors.

Preparation Time: 1 hour

10: Spinach and Feta Stuffed Portobello Mushrooms

Ingredients:

- 4 large portobello mushrooms, stems removed
- 2 cups fresh spinach leaves
- 1/2 cup crumbled feta cheese
- 2 cloves garlic, minced
- 2 tablespoons olive oil
- Salt and pepper to taste
- Balsamic glaze for drizzling

Instructions:

- Preheat the oven to 375°F (190°C). Line a baking sheet with parchment paper.
- In a skillet, heat olive oil over medium heat.
- Add minced garlic and sauté until fragrant.
- Add fresh spinach leaves to the skillet and cook until wilted.
- Remove from heat and stir in crumbled feta cheese. Season with salt and pepper to taste.

> Place portobello mushrooms on the prepared baking sheet.

> Divide the spinach and feta mixture evenly among the mushrooms, filling the caps.

> Bake for 20-25 minutes until mushrooms are tender.

> Drizzle with balsamic glaze before serving.

Health Benefits:

> Portobello mushrooms are low in calories and rich in vitamins and minerals, while spinach and feta cheese provide additional nutrients and flavor, making this dish a nutritious and satisfying dinner option for seniors.

Preparation Time: 30 minutes

Vegetarian Sjogren Syndrome Diet Snacks Recipes

1: Hummus and Veggie Sticks

Ingredients:

> 1/2 cup hummus

> Assorted vegetable sticks (carrots, cucumbers, bell peppers)

Instructions:

> Place hummus in a bowl.
> Wash and cut vegetables into sticks.
> Serve vegetable sticks with hummus for dipping.

Health Benefits:

> Hummus provides plant-based protein and fiber, while vegetables offer vitamins, minerals, and antioxidants, supporting overall health and digestion.

Preparation Time: 5 minutes

2: Greek Yogurt with Honey and Almonds

Ingredients:

> 1/2 cup Greek yogurt
> 1 tablespoon honey
> 1 tablespoon chopped almonds

Instructions:

> Place Greek yogurt in a bowl.
> Drizzle honey over the yogurt.
> Sprinkle chopped almonds on top.

Health Benefits:

> Greek yogurt is rich in protein and probiotics, while honey and almonds provide antioxidants and healthy fats, supporting gut health and immunity.

Preparation Time: 5 minutes

3: Edamame

Ingredients:

> 1 cup cooked edamame (shelled)
> Salt to taste

Instructions:

> Cook edamame according to package instructions.
> Drain and sprinkle with salt.
> Serve as a nutritious snack.
> Health Benefits: Edamame is a good source of plant-based protein, fiber, and essential nutrients, promoting satiety and supporting muscle health.

Preparation Time: 10 minutes

4: Cottage Cheese and Pineapple

Ingredients:

- 1/2 cup cottage cheese
- 1/2 cup diced pineapple

Instructions:

- Place cottage cheese in a bowl.
- Top with diced pineapple.

Health Benefits:

- Cottage cheese is high in protein and calcium, while pineapple provides vitamin C and digestive enzymes, supporting bone health and digestion.

Preparation Time: 5 minutes

5: Rice Cake with Almond Butter and Banana Slices

Ingredients:

- 1 rice cake
- 1 tablespoon almond butter
- 1/2 banana, sliced

Instructions:

> Spread almond butter on the rice cake.
> Top with banana slices.

Health Benefits:

> This snack is a balanced combination of carbohydrates, healthy fats, and vitamins, providing energy and satiety.

Preparation Time: 3 minutes

6: Trail Mix

Ingredients:

> 1/4 cup almonds
> 1/4 cup walnuts
> 1/4 cup dried cranberries
> 1/4 cup pumpkin seeds

Instructions:

> Mix all ingredients together in a bowl.
> Store in an airtight container for a convenient snack.

Health Benefits:

> ➢ Trail mix is a nutrient-dense snack rich in protein, healthy fats, and antioxidants, providing sustained energy and supporting heart health.

Preparation Time: 5 minutes

7: Avocado Rice Crackers

Ingredients:

> ➢ 2 rice crackers
> ➢ 1/2 avocado, mashed
> ➢ Sprinkle of black sesame seeds

Instructions:

> ➢ Spread mashed avocado on rice crackers.
> ➢ Sprinkle black sesame seeds on top.

Health Benefits:

> ➢ Avocado provides healthy fats and fiber, while rice crackers offer a gluten-free and low-calorie base, making this snack satisfying and nutritious.

Preparation Time: 5 minutes

Ingredients:

- Nori seaweed sheets
- Cooked sushi rice
- Assorted thinly sliced vegetables (cucumber, carrot, avocado)
- Soy sauce for dipping

Instructions:

- Place a nori sheet on a bamboo sushi mat.
- Spread a layer of sushi rice on the nori sheet.
- Arrange thinly sliced vegetables on top of the rice.
- Roll the sushi tightly using the bamboo mat.
- Slice into bite-sized pieces and serve with soy sauce.

Health Benefits:

- Veggie sushi rolls are low in calories and rich in vitamins, minerals, and antioxidants, supporting overall health and providing a satisfying snack option.

Preparation Time: 20 minutes

9: Fruit Salad with Mint Yogurt Dressing

Ingredients:

- ➢ Assorted fresh fruits (berries, melon, grapes)
- ➢ 1/2 cup Greek yogurt
- ➢ 1 tablespoon honey
- ➢ Fresh mint leaves, chopped

Instructions:

- ➢ Wash and cut fruits into bite-sized pieces.
- ➢ In a bowl, mix Greek yogurt, honey, and chopped mint leaves to make the dressing.
- ➢ Drizzle the dressing over the fruit salad and toss gently to coat.

Health Benefits:

- ➢ Fruit salad provides vitamins, minerals, and antioxidants, while the mint yogurt dressing adds creaminess and flavor without added sugars.

Preparation Time: 10 minutes

10: Roasted Chickpeas

Ingredients:

- ➤ 1 can chickpeas, drained and rinsed
- ➤ 1 tablespoon olive oil
- ➤ 1 teaspoon ground cumin
- ➤ 1/2 teaspoon smoked paprika
- ➤ Salt to taste

Instructions:

- ➤ Preheat the oven to 400°F (200°C).
- ➤ Pat dry chickpeas with a paper towel and place on a baking sheet.
- ➤ Drizzle with olive oil and sprinkle with ground cumin, smoked paprika, and salt. Toss to coat evenly.
- ➤ Roast in the oven for 20-25 minutes, shaking the pan halfway through, until chickpeas are golden and crispy.
- ➤ Allow to cool before serving.

Health Benefits:

> ➢ Roasted chickpeas are a crunchy and flavorful snack high in protein, fiber, and essential nutrients, supporting satiety and digestive health.

Preparation Time: 30 minutes

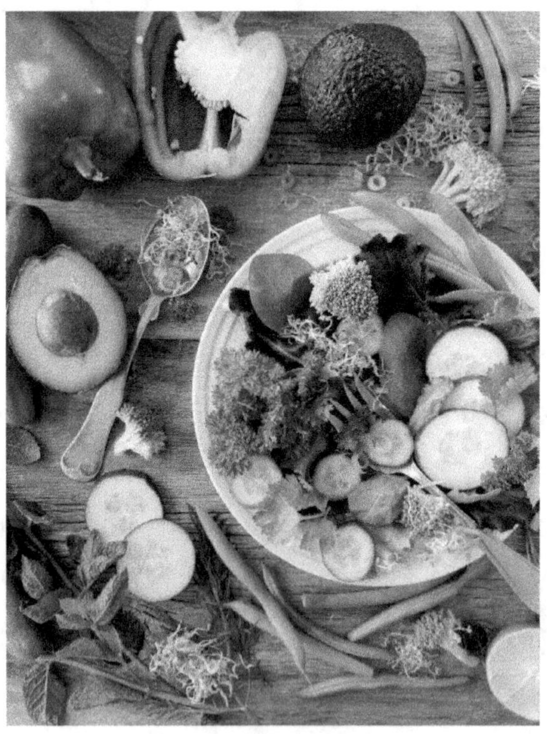

CONCLUSION

The Vegetarian Sjogren Syndrome Diet Cookbook for Seniors offers a comprehensive and practical guide to navigating the dietary challenges presented by this autoimmune condition.

By embracing a plant-based approach rich in hydrating fruits and vegetables, nutrient-dense whole foods, and omega-3 fatty acids, seniors can effectively manage symptoms and promote their overall health and well-being.

Through a collection of easy-to-follow recipes, tailored meal plans, and valuable nutritional guidance, this cookbook empowers seniors with Sjogren's syndrome to make informed choices that support their unique dietary needs.

From nourishing breakfast options to satisfying snacks and hearty main courses, each recipe is thoughtfully crafted to deliver both flavor and functionality.

Moreover, this cookbook emphasizes the importance of consulting with healthcare professionals, including registered dietitians, to personalize dietary recommendations and ensure they align with individual health goals and treatment plans.

With the Vegetarian Sjogren Syndrome Diet Cookbook for Seniors as a trusted resource, seniors can embark on a journey towards improved symptom management, enhanced hydration, and a renewed sense of vitality.

By prioritizing nutritious, plant-based meals, seniors can savor the benefits of a diet designed to nourish both body and soul, supporting them in living their best lives, one delicious bite at a time.